39 HEALTHY TEAS
You Can Make at Home

Mama Prepper

The purpose of this book is to give everyone a chance to stay healthy without depending on the $400 billion pharmaceutical industry.

The next book in this series, *Healing Herbs from Your Kitchen*, is also available.

Additional books in this series are:

Mama Prepper's Herbal Garden

Mama's Medicines – Growing Your Backyard Apothecary

Contents

BIG PHARMA IS POISONING YOU

For thousands of years, people depended upon a variety of teas to stay healthy. They grew herbs in their gardens, served them with their foods, and drank them in their teas.

But the pharmaceutical industry changed all of that. Aspirin, once called a miracle drug, became one of the first culprits. Let's take a closer look at aspirin.

Acetylsalicylic acid, the active ingredient in a number of plants, but most specifically in the inner bark of the willow, is the chemical we now call aspirin. People used the willow in a tea to help with arthritis, sore muscles, headaches, in the same way we take an aspirin today.

Yet we don't use aspirin the way our ancestors used willow bark. Furthermore, many people seem to be sensitive to aspirin. Was that always the case? What may have changed?

While we can't return to the past and research the percentage of people who used to be sensitive to tea made from the bark of the willow, we can follow some basic logic.

When the pharmaceutical industry makes a new drug, they find the active ingredient, isolate it, then synthesize it and patent it. That's how they make their $400 billion dollars each year. So far, that doesn't sound too bad, does it?

What happens next, however, is the problem. Aspirin, in the form of a nice, neat little pill, is so concentrated it punches your stomach lining so hard that taken too frequently will literally punch a hole in your stomach, can cause internal bleeding, and even death.

Those are called "side effects," and all drugs have them, because all drugs are missing the buffering, complimentary, and helping parts that the original source, a plant, has. What that means is that the potent concentration of the active ingredient, isolated from the whole package of the plant, is not something your body handles well. Willow bark, for example, diffused in a cup of water as a tea, is far gentler to your stomach lining. You can, of course, develop a sensitivity to willow bark tea just like you can with aspirin, but it takes far more cups of tea than it does individual aspirin pills.

So, why am I so upset with Big Pharma? The short answer is, they tried to poison me, and had been, in fact, giving me a drug that would produce yet another complicated condition. Their $400 billion-dollar industry is based on keeping us sick and providing us with "cures" that only lead to other conditions that require their services. They are not in the business of getting us healthy. They want us to depend on them for our well-being, and they're the ones who train our doctors.

I am not against doctors. If I have an appendix attack, I want a doctor to do surgery and remove that diseased part of my body, but many of the pills we take as various remedies could very well be unnecessary.

I'm suggesting another way. Here are some teas designed to get you on your way to better health. Some of them you can grow in your garden, or even inside your home. Some are no more than a grocery store away. Many are things you may already have on hand.

INTRODUCTION

Our kitchens are far more pharmaceutical than we realize. Right at our fingertips we have cold and cough medicines, arthritis aids, blood sugar controls, help for high cholesterol, allergy relievers, high blood pressure assistance and even cancer preventatives. We have Power Foods in our refrigerators and on our shelves. We even have remedies for women's issues, such as painful periods.

Although people used to use teas to get and stay healthy, we have all but lost that art. I hope to remedy that.

This particular book will give you a number of herbal teas that will address many of our health issues, complete with instructions in how to prepare them.

**You Can Make These in The Comfort
of Your Own Home**

1
Anise

Anise Seed is a delicious herb that has been around for thousands of years. It tastes great in a number of dishes, including home-made brown bread. The hint of licorice gives the bread a bit of an unexpected kick. Anise Seed is also great in meat dishes.

Anise has a host of medicinal benefits, being rich in antioxidants, vitamins C and A, and minerals such as calcium, coper, iron manganese, magnesium and potassium. Potassium is an important component in helping to control heart rate and blood pressure.

Anise Tea addresses several issues, such as coughs, colds and baby's colic. It promotes mother's milk. A cup of Anise Tea before bed will help you sleep better.

Anise Tea

1 teaspoon crushed Anise Seed
1 cup (approximately) boiling water
Pour water into cup with Anise Seed. (I use a tea ball.)

Let steep 10-20 minutes. Add honey to taste, if desired. Sip slowly.
Delicious!

2
Basil

Who doesn't have a little Basil on hand? If you love pizza, spaghetti and lasagna dishes, it's probably because of the Basil added to the sauce. What a fun and delicious way to get healthy!

As a medicine, Basil addresses a number of issues. It is an anti-inflammatory (think arthritis), it lowers blood sugar (think diabetes), and it lowers cholesterol (think heart disease).

Basil Tea

1 teaspoon dried Basil (or 2 teaspoons fresh)
1 cup boiling water (approximately)
Pour water into the cup with the Basil. (I use a tea ball.)
Strain. Let steep for 10-20 minutes.
Sip slowly.

3

Bay Leaf

Bay leaves are terrific in stews, soups, on meat and to season game. It takes out the "gamey" taste of venison, for example.

As a medicine, it works against gastrointestinal issues such as ulcers, digestive complaints, diarrhea, and flatulence. It's even gentle enough for baby's colic.

Drink a cup of Bay Leaf Tea in the evening.

Bay Leaf Tea

1 Bay Leaf
1 cup boiling water

Pour water over Bay leaf. Let sit for about 10 minutes.

This tea is mild and can be used for infants with colic.

As a fever reducer, you will be pleasantly surprised

at how well it works. It also eases the muscle aches of the flu, and fights the congestion of bronchitis from a cold. As a pain reliever, it works to ease arthritis and muscle aches.

Other Uses

Teas aren't just used for drinking. If you add a little salt, you can use it as a gargle for a sore throat at any time during the day.

For additional help during the flu season, soak a cloth that has been soaked in boiled Bay leaves and water, and place on the chest as a compress.

4

California Poppy

There are times when a person needs a preventative for convulsions or muscle spasms, such as febrile seizures, which are more common in infants and small children. If they have this tendency, their fevers can spike within minutes from just above normal to 105 degrees or more. If you have a child with this tendency, every time they become sick, dose them with some Strong California Poppy Tea. All above-ground parts can be used.

Strong California Poppy Tea

2 teaspoons dried California Poppy flowers, stems, leaves and/or seeds.
1 cup boiling water
Pour boiling water over dried California Poppy
Let steep 10 minutes.
May sweeten to taste.

May drink 1-2 cups daily while needed.

5

Caraway

The reason plants work so well for health is that for them to survive, they need to have natural protections against bugs and diseases. We call those protections medicines.

Many of these herbs work against digestive distress. Caraway is one of these herbs. Caraway Tea can relieve gas and increase kidney strength. Used with other meds, it can reduce nausea and stomach cramps. A mild caraway tea even works on colic.

Mild Caraway Tea

Boil 1 teaspoon of Caraway Seeds in 1-2 liters of water for 15 minutes.

Strain.

May be served either hot or warm. Babies, of course, prefer it barely warm, and sweetened with a touch of honey.

6

Cayenne

Every garden should grow some cayenne. Not only is it a terrific spice, but it's a fine medicine. If you suffer from a cold, sore throat, cough, or a digestive complaint, drink a little Cayenne Medicinal Tea.

Cayenne Medicinal Tea.

1/8th teaspoon to 1 cup water

Mix well and drink (or gargle if for laryngitis)

Works as a mouthwash too.

7

Chamomile

Chamomile is every tea-lover's favorite. This soothing anti-inflammatory tea can be sipped before bed to ease sore muscles into relaxing so that you can get to sleep easier. It's also a gentle anxiety reliever for those difficult days when there were too many worries and not enough solutions. Encourage your mind to relax with a cup of Chamomile Tea.

Chamomile Tea

1 teaspoon dried Chamomile flowers (or 2 teaspoons fresh)
1 cup boiling water
Pour water over flowers.
Let steep 10 minutes, or longer if you prefer a slightly bitter flavor.
Strain. Add honey to taste, if desired.
Sip slowly.

8

Chives

Chives are one of those plants you can keep on your kitchen windowsill. They winter over well, but you will want to keep a fresh supply on hand. Fresher is always better when it comes to plants. Chives help prevent cancer by inhibiting the growth of tumors. It has been used in treating esophageal, stomach, prostate and gastrointestinal track cancers.

Most of us, however, don't think of preventing cancer when we drink tea, so consider cancer prevention a pleasant side effect. Chives are an excellent source of anti-bacterials and a source for heart health.

Chive Tea

You will want to play around with the strength of this tea. Chives are a part of the onion family, and although milder than their cousins have a taste that must be acquired.

1 teaspoon chopped Chive tops
1 cup (approximately) boiling water

Pour water over chive tops (I use a tea ball).
Let steep for about 10-20 minutes. Strain.
Sip slowly and enjoy.

9
Cinnamon

If it were possible to grow my own cinnamon, I would. This lovely spice gives teas, oatmeal, breads and desserts an amazing flavor. But as a medicine, none is its equal. It works to ease the aches of arthritis. Drink this tasty tea up to three times a day.

Arthritis Tea

1 cup hot water
2 teaspoons Honey
1 teaspoon Cinnamon

Mix together and drink three times a day to ease arthritis pain.

Now for an amazing bonus, how to address bladder infections. Who gets bladder infections? Newlywed women do. This isn't talked about very often, but because of the frequency of sex, sometimes bacteria gets pushed into the urethra causing a bladder infection. So do those who don 't drink enough water. Dehydration causes the bladder to be unable to eliminate toxins effectively, making bladder infections more likely.

Bladder Infection Tea

1 cup warm water
2 tablespoons Cinnamon
1 teaspoon Honey
Mix together.

Drink once per day until urine runs clear.

10

Cilantro

Are you looking for an all-purpose herb? Cilantro is one of those no medicine chest should be without. It is essential in Mexican dishes, but also makes a pleasant-tasting tea that addresses a variety of conditions.

Do you have allergies? Unless you are allergic to Cilantro, a tea made with either leaves or seeds have an antihistamine effect.

Have you recently eaten something that made you sick? Cilantro contains high levels of a natural antibiotic that counteracts deadly salmonella food poisoning. So if you suspect the food being served, eat some salsa with Cilantro in it. If you're already sick from food poisoning, sip some Mild Cilantro Tea.

Being high in iron, cilantro also addresses anemia. High in calcium, cilantro assists bone health. Because it contains natural antibiotics and antivirals, cilantro works well against all kinds disorders, colds, flu, and other viruses.

Cilantro regulates secretions from the endocrine glands, and regulates hormones. As a result, it can regulate periods, and even reduce the associated pain.

Are you diabetic? Drink Strong Cilantro Tea daily to help regulate blood sugar.

However, you can also use Strong Cilantro Tea as a topical, applying it to cuts and sores, because it's a wonderful antibiotic. It also works on skin inflammation, against fungi, and to ease eczema.

Mild Cilantro Tea

1 cup boiling water
1 teaspoon Cilantro leaves and seeds
Pour water over seeds and let steep 10-20 minutes.
Sip slowly.

Strong Cilantro Tea

1 tablespoon Cilantro leaves and seeds
2 to 4 cups boiling water
Boil together for five minutes. Let steep for 5-14 minutes longer. Strain.
Sip slowly.

11
Cloves

Cloves are another powerhouse seed. You might think of it as a Super Spice with more antioxidants, more antiseptic, more germicidal, and more anti-inflammatory properties than most of your kitchen herbs.

If you are fighting arthritis pain, and if you have high blood pressure, this is the spice for you.

Clove Tea

1 cup boiling water (approximately)
1/4 teaspoon Clove powder
Honey to taste
Let steep about 10-20 minutes. Strain.

OR:

Add 1/4 teaspoon Clove powder to another hot beverage, such as hot apple juice, green tea, or spiced tea. It is scrumptious with hot apple juice!

12
Cornflower

Cornflower is also called Bachelor Buttons. They seed themselves down, so plant them where you want them to grow permanently. They can be blue, lavender, pink and white. Some find them "weedy" looking, but I like them. Just think, you never have to replant.

Eye Medicine

If you have an eye condition or inflammation, an infusion made of the leaves of the plant can help. Make a Mild Cornflower Leaf Tea and let cool completely. Put one or two drops in the affected eye twice a day.

Tired Eyes

If you are suffering from tired eyes, pour boiling water over fresh or dried flowers. Put in refrigerator. Apply chilled flowers to closed eyes and rest for a while.

Mild Cornflower Leaf Tea

1 teaspoon dried cornflower leaves

1 cup boiling water
Pour water over dried leaves.
Let steep about 10 minutes
May add mint or honey to taste.
Sip slowly.
For an eyewash, let cool completely.

Energizer

The dried flower petals are useful for energizing and stimulating the body. Just make a Mild Cornflower Petal Tea and slip slowly. The tea will be bitter. You may also add mint or honey to taste.

Mild Cornflower Petal Tea

1 teaspoon dried Cornflower Petals
1 cup boiling water
Pour water over dried petals. (May also add mint.)
Let steep for 10 minutes or longer.
Sip slowly.
May add honey to taste.

Digestion

If you have digestive problems, a little leaf or flower tea, or the two combined, may solve the issue. For the most part, the flowers are the most common part of Cornflower to be used.

Detoxifying Liver

If you are overweight, your liver will need help (you're making it do too much) and may need a boost. This is when a Mild Cornflower Petal Tea (see above) could be beneficial to your health. How would you know? If your doctor says you can't take NSAIDS (Aleve, Ibuprofen, aspirin and the like) any longer, you have a damaged liver. Losing weight is your best solution (difficult, I know), along with a daily dose of detoxifying tea.

Resist Infection

If you get a wound or scrape, you can wash the injury with a Strong Cornflower Tea as an antiseptic.

Strong Cornflower Tea

2 teaspoons dried Cornflower Petals
1 cup boiling water
Pour water over petals.
Let steep for about 10 minutes.
Add honey to taste, if desired.
Sip slowly.

Mild Baby Laxative

The best parts of Cornflower to use for a baby laxative are the seeds.

To make **Mild Baby Laxative Tea**:

1 teaspoon crushed Cornflower seeds
1 cup boiling water
Pour water over seeds.
Let steep about 10 minutes.
Strain into cup.

Add a touch of honey if desired.
Allow baby to drink as much or as little as the child wants.

Rheumatic Disorders

Although rheumatism is only used colloquially, as there is no specific disease such as rheumatism, it often refers to chronic joint and muscle issues such as arthritis. It's nice to know there is something to ease the pain. The leaves of the Cornflower, either dried or fresh, have been used in teas for that exact purpose. I would add a little mint, which is also a mild analgesic, to my Cornflower Leaf Tea.

Cornflower Leaf Tea

1 teaspoon fresh or dried Cornflower leaves (plus Mint, if you desire)
1 cup boiling water
Pour water over leaves.
Let steep about 10 minutes.
Strain.
Sip slowly. (honey to taste, optional)

Astringent

The purpose of an astringent is to dry up a skin condition, such as acne or an oozing wound. A mild Cornflower tea, using either leaves, petals, or both, makes an excellent astringent. Allow the tea to cool. If you keep the tea in the refrigerator, it becomes re-freshing as well. Cornflower tea helps stop bleeding too.

Promotes Menstruation

Not every woman has this problem, but I did as a young woman. I would suffer from very painful menstruation because my uterus had trouble holding a full menstrual flow. The issue corrected itself after my first pregnancy. I lost the baby, but it did stretch my uterus enough that I never had those debilitating menstrual pains again. I wish I had known about Cornflower Tea then.

Anyway, if you, also, have trouble with excessive bloating and pain during your menstrual cycle, sip on some Cornflower tea. Added Mint is good with this.

13

Dandelion Leaf

Dandelions mean more than Dandelion Wine or a Spring Tonic. Dandelions, especially the tasty spring dandelions that are not bitter, are good for you. Loaded with Vitamins A, C, D, and B, dandelion tea can actually feed you.

Dandelion Tea

1 teaspoon dried Dandelion Leaves (or 2 teaspoons fresh)
1 cup boiling water
Pour water over leaves. Let steep 10-20 minutes.
Strain. Add honey to taste, if desired.
Sip slowly.

14
Dill

Dill is far more than just the spice you put in pickles to give them that lovely dill flavor. Dill fights osteoporosis, arthritis and painful menstruation. Its stems, leaves and seed heads are high in calcium, which helps to mend broken bones. To address osteoporosis, drink a Strong Dill Tea twice daily.

It is also an anti-inflammatory, making it useful for arthritis and painful menstruation.

Strong Dill Tea

2 teaspoons crushed Dill seeds
1 cup boiling water
Pour water over crushed Dill seed.

15
Echinacea

It's a beautiful flower. Plant a lot of them, and let them grow, because it's the root you need as a medicine. They'll seed down, and because they can be prolific, you don't need to feel guilty by harvesting the roots in the second year once they've become established.

Echinacea Anti-Inflammatory Tea

1 teaspoon dried and ground Echinacea Root
1 cup boiling water
Pour water over dried root.
Let steep 30 minutes
As a topical remedy, apply an echinacea cloth directly to affected area or as a tea take 1 tablespoon of liquid 3-6 times per day.

Analgesic

If you are sensitive to NSAIDS, you could try Echinacea as a substitute pain-killer in the place of Willow-bark Tea, for example, which is the origin of aspirin. As stated above, the parts used are the leaves and roots.

Echinacea Anti-Inflammatory Tea is a good NSAID substitute.

The Tea also works for sore throats, including strep infections.

Antiviral

Flu and colds are viruses. Yes, there are plants that can fight viruses, including AIDS, covid and all its variants. Echinacea is a natural anti-viral, which is why it has become known as a cold and flu fighter.

When you first feel the signs of a cold or flu coming on, take Echinacea Anti-Inflammatory Tea 6 times per day for 2-3 days, then taper off to twice a day for the remainder of the infection.

Antibacterial

Viruses aren't the only "bugs" that attack human bodies. Echinacea is also an excellent antibacterial.

You can use the **Echinacea Anti-Inflammatory Tea** as an antibacterial wash. Apply to affected area with clean cloth or cotton ball.

Antiseptic

Do you want help in keeping your sickroom clean, or in cleaning wounds and abrasions? Your answer might be in using an antiseptic wash made with **Echinacea Anti-Inflammatory Tea.**

If the problem is an infected wound, sore, boil, abrasion, you can make an ointment with fresh Echinacea Leaves, or a tincture made with Echinacea Root.

Echinacea is also a folk remedy for the **brown recluse spider** bite. Catch it early. Apply any of the topical Echinacea remedies for the bite, the Tea, Ointment, Tincture or Salve.

16
Fennel

Fennel has a yellow seed head very much like Dill, but there the comparison ends. Fennel is its own food and herb, and a must-have for any garden.

Fennel Tea:

1 teaspoon Fennel seeds
1 cup boiling water
Pour water over crushed seeds. Let steep for 10-15 minutes. Sip slowly.

Fennel Tea helps to settle a too-rich meal, settle indigestion, and cures flatulence. It is common practice in some parts of the world to chew a few seeds after each meal to aid in digestion and freshen the breath.

Clean a Sick Room

To clean the sickroom, boil the leaves, and wash all surfaces with Fennel water.

Respiratory Ailments

Fennel tea with honey makes an excellent tea for coughs and bronchitis because it has expectorant qualities. Crush dried Fennel leaves into a powder and place in a gelatin capsule when drinking a tea is not available. The properties in Fennel help to break up congestion and phlegm, and work to cleanse the body of the toxins that cause respiratory ailments.

Eye Care

Fennel protects against inflammation. A weak fennel tea, thoroughly strained, can be used as an eye wash for treating conjunctivitis in infected eyes. In addition, fresh Fennel leaves can be made into a cold compress to be applied over the eyes to reduce irritation and eye fatigue. Its overall health properties in keeping skin cells, blood wall cells and others, also keep eye tissue healthy.

Facial

While steeping your Fennel Tea, bend over the steam, with a cloth tented around you, and breathe in the steam. It will open your pores and rejuvenate your facial skin.

17
Feverfew

Feverfew gets its name from it's ability to reduce fevers and inflammation. But it has a host of other benefits. It helps your body reduce flatulence (gas), including the bloating that comes right before and during menses. It works as a mild laxative, fights parasites, and more, but DO NOT TAKE IF PREGNANT.

Flatulence

Along with gas often comes stomach upsets. For digestive issues, including colic, make a Mild Feverfew Tea. This also works as a tonic.

Mild Feverfew Tea

1 scant teaspoon dried Feverfew flowers, leaves and bark
1 cup boiling water
Pour water over herb.
Let steep about 10 minutes.
May add honey to taste.
Sip slowly.

Promoting Menstruation

Many women suffer from the bloating and discomfort of painful menses. Feverfew can relieve this discomfort. Also, if your period is delayed, Mild Feverfew Tea can help.

But do not take this if you're pregnant. Mild Feverfew Tea can also cause uterine contractions.

DO NOT TAKE IF PREGNANT

Laxative

If you need relief from constipation, a cup of Mild Feverfew Tea might be the answer. Don't be busy while you sip your tea. Sometimes we are constipated because we are too busy, and our body is getting the message that we aren't doing this right now. So relax and enjoy a few moments of stillness.

Reducing Fever

Feverfew has been used to reduce fevers. It may not work as well as people once thought, however, since it is also an anti-inflammatory, it may work against the things that *cause* fevers instead. If you're running a fever, you may take a Mild Feverfew Tea up to four times a day.

Anti-Inflammatory

If you are taking Feverfew for migraines, you may find that your rheumatoid arthritis pain is diminishing as well. This is a welcome side-effect for arthritis sufferers. Feverfew is a natural anti-inflammatory. You may take Mild Feverfew Tea up to four times per day.

18
Garlic

Every house should have garlic in the kitchen, garlic powder, granules, or fresh, it doesn't matter. Garlic is far more than just a tasty addition to food. Garlic is a potent medicine, especially when you're coming down with a cold. That tiny tickle or dry spot in the back of your throat that drinking a glass water doesn't quite fix, that's when you drink some garlic tea. You drink it for three days. Your symptoms will disappear in the first day, and you'll think it was your imagination, that you really weren't coming down with a cold after all, but drink it two more days anyway. Your chances of avoiding that cold altogether just increased tremendously.

Garlic Tea (if you already have a sore throat)

Steep several cloves of Garlic in 1/2 cup of water overnight.
In morning, hold nose to drink it, unless the smell doesn't bother you.
Let cool, then strain into bottle and cap tightly.

Garlic Tea (for that tickle I mentioned in the introduction)

Crush one dried clove.
Put in a cup.
Add boiling water (and a little basil for flavor, if you wish.)
Sip slowly.

19

Ginger

When I was a young woman, my husband's grand-mother gave me a cup of ginger tea for my cramps. This was my first introduction to herbal remedies. Previously, I had always used ginger in cookies and pies. Ginger boosts circulation, eases nausea, and soothes morning sickness in pregnant women.

Ginger Tea

Slice 3 to five thin slices from a fresh ginger root. Place in boiling water for 3 minutes (the amount of water is up to you).
Steep for 3 minutes. Strain. Add honey, if desired. Sip slowly to let the ginger work its magic.

However, my husband's grandmother just put a half a teaspoon of powdered ginger from a spice jar in a cup of hot water. My, that was good!

20
Goldenseal Root

If you've been sick and cannot seem to get well, you may take a Goldenseal Root Tea by the tablespoon throughout the day. This is not a tea you sip with a meal, or to relax. Never take more than 1 cup in any given day. Discontinue use after three weeks. Discontinue use if you develop mouth sores or any other side-effects. Give your body a minimum two-week rest before trying this remedy again.

Goldenseal Root Tea

1 teaspoon chopped, dried Goldenseal Root
1 cup boiling water
Pour water over chopped, dried herb.
Let sit until cool.
Strain.
Take liquid by tablespoonful throughout the day.
Discontinue use after 3 weeks.

Parasites

Goldenseal Root Tea will also rid the body of internal

parasites. Make the tea as directed above, and take no more than 1 tablespoon at a time, drinking no more than 1 cup per day.

Colds, Bronchitis

Because of its antibacterial/antiviral effects, Goldenseal Root Tea helps fight colds and flu, and a variety of other viral infections.

Make some Goldenseal Root Tea (see above). Take no more than 1 cup per day, a tablespoon at a time throughout the day.

Stomach Complaints

Goldenseal Root Tea also works for ulcers and other stomach complaints. It is a bitter herb that stimulates bile. It has been used to stop diarrhea.

Make some Goldenseal Root Tea (see above). Take no more than 1 cup per day, a tablespoon at a time throughout the day.

Eye Infections

As an eyewash for pink eye and other eye infections, Goldenseal Root Tea works well here too. Follow instructions on the above recipes.

Cautions:

Goldenseal is not for long-term use.

Goldenseal should not be used by pregnant women

or by children under two.

Goldenseal may cause stomach irritations, especially when taken for too long.

Do not take Goldenseal if you have high blood pressure.

21
Green Tea

Are you under stress? Have you recently moved, gotten a divorce, suffered the death of a loved one, started back to school, made a job change, or any other major change in your life? If so, you are under stress, even if any of those things were right to do. There are a number of other stresses in life as well, living through chaotic times, dealing with difficult people, whether co-workers or family. Many things put stress in our lives.

And stress can make us sick. So what can we do about it?

Drink green tea!

Aside from helping your body deal with stress, Green Tea has been used for:

- Cancer
- Prevent Tooth Decay
- Immune System
- Sunburn
- High Blood Pressure

- Lower Blood Sugar

Cancer

Properties in green tea have been proven to destroy free radicals. It is also full of antioxidants. One in particular, "EGCG," has been proven to reduce tumor growth.

Green Tea is a wonderful anti-cancer medication. It can slow, and sometimes even stop, the growth of cancer cells. It has been shown to help defeat lung cancer. Of course, that does not mean if you drink Green Tea while you smoke a cigarette, you'll be safe. Nothing can cure such stupidity. But Green Tea can be your front line of defense.

Prevent Tooth Decay

Green Tea has antibacterial agents that can keep you healthy. These agents have been known to slow the growth of dental plaque.

Immune System

Because of these agents, drinking green tea stimulates the immune system and fights infection.

Sunburn

Applying it directly to skin after a sunburn can even help rejuvenate skin and promote quicker healing. It will even attack skin cancer cells that may be forming on your skin if you spend a lot of time under the sun.

High Blood Pressure

Green tea is a mild diuretic. As a result it can lower high blood pressure. It helps with high cholesterol too by destroying bad cholesterol and promoting good cholesterol.

I drink green tea every morning with a little lemon. The lemon is good for lowering blood pressure too.

Blood Sugar

Diabetics rejoice. Drinking green tea can lower your blood sugar. Drink 2-3 cups a day for maximum effect.

That is really good news! With so many benefits and only one caution, how can you lose?

One caution: Those with overactive thyroid should be cautious using green tea.

22

Hawthorn

If you have room for trees in your garden or your yard, you might want to consider a Hawthorn Tree. The leaves, flowers and berries can all be used medicinally.

Digestive Aid

Take a cup of Mild Hawthorn Tea as a digestive aid, especially after too much, or too rich an evening meal.

Mild Hawthorn Tea

Although a tea can be made with the leaves, flowers and berries of the tree, it depends on the time of year which parts you will be using for your tea. One solution is to dry some leaves and flowers for making Mild Hawthorn Tea throughout the year.

When the berries are ripe, dry the berries as well for later use. I would use the berries for **heart conditions and as a detoxifier**. It works especially well for heart problems, but do not take longer than three months at a time, and no more than two teaspoons in a day.

1 teaspoon dried leaves and flowers
1 cup boiling water
Pour water over leaves and flowers.
Let steep about 10 minutes.
Strain.
Sip slowly.
May add honey to taste.

Sore Throats

For a sore throat, the dried berries, leaves and flowers can be used in your Mild Hawthorn Tea. For a sore throat, be sure to add the honey.

Tonic

To get the maximum benefit of Hawthorn, take as a tonic daily for no more than three months, then discontinue for at least two months. A tonic is a tea, most often with a mixture of cleansing herbs that heal the liver. The liver is the body's primary cleansing organ. It takes quite a bit of abuse throughout our lifetime, especially if a person is taking prescription medications. So if an herb is identified as a detoxifier, you now know that the part of the body that it is detoxifying is the liver. Take a tonic in the spring, during the winter, or after an illness.

23
Hibiscus

If you have ever sipped Celestial Seasonings' Red Zinger, then you have an idea of the taste of Hibiscus Tea. This beautiful, red sour tea is a great summertime drink. But if you like it in the summer, you may want to drink it all year once you discover how healthy it is.

Like many plants, Hibiscus has natural antibacterial, anticancer and astringent properties. The astringent properties mean it will work as a diuretic, just like coffee and black tea. It also has mild laxative properties. This doesn't mean it will give you the runs necessarily, but it will help if you have constipation problems because of medication or diet.

Parts used: flower, fruit and calyx (the cup that holds the petals and the fruit). Although all three parts are used for medicinal purposes, it's the calyx that are used the most.

Hibiscus has been used for:

- High Blood Pressure and High Cholesterol
- Sleep Aid
- Nutrition
- Weight Loss

High Blood Pressure and High Cholesterol

In some recent studies, Hibiscus was shown to reduce both. Hibiscus Tea could be included as part of your daily diet to help control both of these issues. You will need to drink several cups a day.

Hibiscus Tea

1 teaspoon dried Hibiscus, crumbled
1 cup boiling water
Pour water over herb
Let steep about 10 minutes
Strain
May had honey to taste
Sip slowly

Sleep Aid Tea

Equal parts of Hibiscus, St. John's Wort and Lemon Balm
1 cup boiling water for every teaspoon of herb mixture
Pour water over herbs
Let steep for about 10 minutes
Strain
May add honey to taste
Sip slowly

Nutrition

Why take C tablets when you can just drink Hibiscus Tea? It's very high in Vitamin C and calcium, and contains natural antioxidants (Vitamin C is one of them).

Weight Loss

Not only is Hibiscus nutritious, but it has the constituent hydroxy citric acid (HCA) from which Hydroxycut, the appetite suppressant, is made. So, drink a cup of Hibiscus Tea, feed yourself and lose weight at the same time!

How to Grow:

The type of Hibiscus you want for tea is *Hibiscus sabdariffa*, which needs a tropical environment to grow. Get plants from your favorite nursery and grow them indoors, if you wish. The bright red calyx is the part used the most for medicinal tea.

Hibiscus Acetosella is not medicinal.

24

Honeysuckle

I love Honeysuckle. It reminds me of my grand-mother's place, with the summer hot and humid, and fragrant with Honeysuckle vines. I also love it for its ability to hide a compost pile or a chicken pen when you live in a city. That it also can be used to relieve headaches is a plus.

Headache

There are many different kinds and causes of head-aches. But when you have one, you aren't looking for the cause, but for quick results. Honeysuckle is a natural anti-inflammatory, so if the cause of your headache is a sinus infection, you'll be pleas-antly surprised with the results. The main attribute of Honeysuckle, however, is its analgesic properties, meaning it relieves pain.

Honeysuckle Tea

Using fresh Honeysuckle, chop up flowers, leaves and stems until you have a small pile of chopped herb.

Use 2 teaspoons of freshly chopped flowers and put in a tea ball or right into your cup.

Add 1 cup boiling water and let steep for 10-20 minutes. The longer you let it steep, the more potent will be your tea.

Strain. Sip slowly.

For Winter Use you can also dry the leaves, stems and flowers and store the dried herbs in jars with tightly fitting lids. In the winter, use 1 teaspoon of Honeysuckle to one cup of water.

25
Horehound

Horehound has been used for thousands of years for colds, coughs, bronchitis and respiratory infections. It hasn't been until recently that horehound drops have been relegated (in this country) to a candy and not a cough remedy. Regardless of the political position of this country, Horehound works. And it works as a tea also.

Respiratory Infections, Coughs, Bronchitis

Horehound has expectorant and antitussive properties. This means that when you have a cold it permits your body to get rid of phlegm as it builds up while it keeping you from bouts of nonproductive spasmodic coughing.

Furthermore, it is an anti-inflammatory and vasodilator, which means it will help to fight lung inflammation while opening the blood vessels so they can work to help the lungs to clear.

Cough drops aren't the only way to take Horehound. If you find that you have a cold, you can make a

Horehound Tea and drink it up to four times per day.

Horehound Tea

1 teaspoon dried or 2 teaspoons fresh Horehound leaves
1 cup boiling water
Pour water over leaves.
Let steep about 10 minutes.
Strain.
Add honey if needed for cough or dry, scratchy throat.
Cover.
Take 1 tablespoon of liquid, as needed.

Sore Throats

There are two ways to address a sore throat with Horehound. One is to take Horehound Tea, sweetened with honey, by the spoonful. The other, of course, is Horehound Drops, and pretend the United States only considers it a candy.

26
Hyssop

Teas can be used as compresses as well. Such is the case with Hyssop when used for bruises, sprains, and burns. You can also drink the tea to address mild anxiety. Hyssop is NOT to be used if you're pregnant.

Bruises and Sprains

There are several ways to use Hyssop to address a bruise or sprain. One is to apply a Hyssop Tea to a cold cloth and apply to the affected area. Then wrap with a long bandage to give the area support as well. May change dressing as often as needed.

Hyssop Tea

1 teaspoon dried Hyssop (2 teaspoons fresh)
1 cup boiling water
Pour water over Hyssop (leaves and flowers).
Let steep for about 10 minutes.
Strain. May sip the tea from the one cup throughout the day.

Cool first if using for a bruise or sprain.

Burns

Apply a rag saturated with Hyssop Tea to the affected area.

Mild Anxiety

Hyssop is a nervine and a mild sedative. Because of its calming effect, Hyssop has been used to calm anxiety. It has also been used to treat those subject to petit mal seizures, a form of epilepsy.

Do not use if pregnant, however.

27

Lantana

When you get a cold, the cough remedy you want is a relaxing expectorant. You want to stop coughing spasms that don't get rid of phlegm, and you do want to expel the balls of phlegm that need to go. Lantana Tea provides that.

Relaxing Expectorant

If you're suffering from a cold or chest congestion, Lantana tea works wonders. It's a relaxing expectorant, which means it helps promote a productive cough while easing the coughing spasms. Just sip a Lantana Tea and let it do its job.

Lantana Tea

2 teaspoons fresh Lantana leaves,
    or 1 teaspoon dried Lantana root
1 cup boiling water
Pour water over leaves.
Let steep about 10 minutes.
Strain.
Sip slowly.

Does your cold or flu include a headache? You could try a Lantana Breathing Steam. This works for sinus and chest congestion too, as well as for breathing problems.

Note: If you want to store Lantana for winter use, *dry the root* for that purpose.

28

Lavender

Even if you never use it for its medicinal properties, Lavender is a lovely herb to grow in your garden. But as a medicine, there is so much you can do with these flowers! They can be used for aromatherapy to reduce headaches and stress. They can be put in your bath, added to home-made soap, in an anti-fungal ointment, as well as a delightful, relaxing tea right before bed.

It can also help with digestive issues, headaches and other aches and pains. As a topical, a cold rag soaked in lavender tea can work wonders.

Lavender Tea

2 teaspoons dried flowers (or 4 teaspoons fresh). Pick the lavender just as the buds are opening for best results.

1 cup boiling water.

Pour water over flowers. Let steep 10-20 minutes. You may or may not want honey to taste in this fragrant beverage.

Breathe in aroma before sipping. Add to your pleasure of enjoying this tea.

29

Lemon Balm

Lemon Balm is a member of the mint family. It has a delightful lemony flavor and goes well when brewed with your black tea for iced tea, a great summertime beverage. But Lemon Balm has other advantages. It inhibits viruses, fights headaches, and reduces insomnia. Best of all, it is well known for helping to treat anxiety, especially when combined with St. John's Wort flowers and leaves.s

Lemon Balm Tea

1-2 teaspoons dried Lemon Balm
1 cup boiling water.
Pour water over leaves.
Let steep 10-20 minutes.
Strain.
Sip slowly.

30
Marjoram

Are you looking for an all-purpose herb that tastes good in food too? You might want to consider Marjoram. It not only fights microbial infections, but it's also a mild analgesic, digestive aid, sinus reliever, and anti-depressant.

Microbial Infections

Marjoram contains antibacterial, antiseptic and antiviral properties. It will address such conditions as food poisoning, and viruses like flu, mumps and measles. It works as a preventative to tetanus. Any time you get a cut, scrape or wound, apply a Mild Marjoram Tea solution to the cut before bandaging.

Marjoram Tea will also work on conditions like malaria (which is a protozoan infection) and typhoid, but the best solution to typhoid is cleanliness. Always boil water 20 minutes before drinking, and keep your environment and your body, especially your hands, clean.

It is also a mild analgesic. So for those who are NSAID sensitive (aspirin-like products, try Marjoram Tea instead.

Mild Marjoram Tea

1 teaspoon dried Marjoram in a cup
Add 1 cup boiling water
Let steep for 10-20 minutes
Can drink 1-4 cups daily
Honey to taste

Indigestion

Make Mild Marjoram Tea. Drink 2 cups over the next two hours slowly.

Mouthwash or Gargle

Make Mild Marjoram Tea, unsweetened, and add a little salt. Cool. Then use as a mouthwash or gargle.

Hay Fever, Sinus Congestion, Asthma, Colds, Coughs (expectorant)

Drink Mild Marjoram Tea as needed.

Digestive Aid

To increase digestion efficiency, calm the stomach, improve appetite, relieve nausea and excessive gas, address intestinal parasites, relieve diarrhea and intestinal infections, relieve constipation and soothe stomach distress, drink a Mild Marjoram Tea , can drink up to 4 cups daily.

Strong Marjoram Tea, Using Fresh Marjoram

Grind fresh Marjoram into paste.
2-6 teaspoons fresh Marjoram paste
Add 1 cup cold water
Let soak for 24 hours
Strain liquid into cup
Add honey

Antidepressant

Use the strongest recipe (6 teaspoons for each cup of water) as an antidepressant and nervous disorders.

31
Oregano

Oregano inhibits the growth of bacteria and other microorganisms, and it tastes delicious! The latest research is finding that Oregano's antibiotic properties parallel those of streptomycin and penicillin. It is an excellent herb for a vaginal or yeast infection. To address these issues, you will need to drink Strong Oregano Tea three times a day.

Strong Oregano Tea
Wash fresh Oregano leave, then chop. Or use dried Oregano.
Put 1 cup chopped Oregano leaves into 4 cups water.
Boil for 15 minutes.
Let steep for 5 minutes.
Strain liquid from leaves.
Drink 1/2 cup three times per day.

32
Parsley

With parsley, either grow your own, or buy it at the store. Don't harvest your parsley in the wild unless you know your herbs. Fool's Parsley can kill you.

That said, Parsley is great for kidney stones, bladder infections and to start delayed menses.

DO NOT USE IF PREGNANT.

For infections and kidney stones, the part of the plant you'll need for this tea is the root.

Parsley Root Tea

2 teaspoons of fresh, chopped Parsley root (1 teaspoon of dried root)
1 cup boiling water
Pour boiling water over Parsley root.
Set steep 10-20 minutes. Strain into cup.
Sip slowly, 1-3 cups a day.

Parsley Leaf Tea

Parsley Leaf Tea is used for a variety of other conditions such as bone health, fighting cancer, eye health, heart health and contains antibacterial properties.

With Parsley, however, your best use is not a tea at all, but to eat it throughout the day, or dry it and add a little to every meal. It's that valuable.

33

Peppermint

Mint's major claim to fame is the way it addresses digestive issues. What you may not know is how extensive this treatment is. Not only does it settle indigestion, but it also works against flatulence, stomach cramps, menstrual cramps, and vomiting.

A terrific bonus for using mint as a daily beverage is that it works as a decongestant and breaks up phlegm. Its active ingredient is menthol.

All of the above is easy with just a little mint tea. You can also add mint to other teas and beverages for an added refreshing taste.

Mint Tea

1 teaspoon dried mint
1 cup boiling water Pour water over dried leaves
Let steep 10-20 minutes.
Strain. May add honey to taste, if desired.
Sip slowly. Let the mint do its job.

34

Raspberry Leaf

We all love raspberries. But did you know that the leaf is just as valuable, if not more so, than the fruit? Raspberry leaves are rich in a host of nutrients that include iron, B vitamin, magnesium and potassium. It has been used to ease menstrual cramps, and to strengthen the uterus and pelvic muscles. It works against diarrhea because of its astringent qualities, and helps alleviate nausea.

DO NOT USE IF PREGNANT

Raspberry Leaf Tea

Always use *dried* Raspberry Leaf.
1 teaspoon dried Raspberry Leaf
1 cup boiling water
Pour water over leaves, and let steep for 5 minutes, then strain.
May drink up to 6 cups per day.

35
Rosehips

Rose hips are the fruit of the rose. They are high in vitamin C, and are a great wintertime nutrient, especially when you can't afford to buy fresh fruits and vegetables. We're spoiled in this country, to have so many foods available all winter long, but it wasn't always so. People used to cherish the rose hip because it prevented scurvy and boosted the immune system, a great advantage during cold and flu season.

Rosehip Tea

Pick your rose hips and dry them. Then take 4 tablespoons of dried rosehips and place in a saucepan. Add 4 cups water. Cover and bring to a boil. Simmer for 5 minutes.

Strain into jar and cool.

When cool enough to drink, pour some into a teacup and enjoy. The remainder may be stored in the refrigerator to enjoy later.

36

Rosemary

In colder climates, you'll want to make Rosemary a part of your indoor garden. This aromatic herb can be added to salads, soups, baked vegetables and breads.

Rosemary helps to detoxify the liver. What happens when a person takes NSAIDS (such as Ibuprofen, Aleve, and a number of other analgesics) for conditions like arthritis, is that it builds up in the liver. The liver handles whole foods like Rosemary better than it does heavy doses of artificial chemicals. Then your doctor will tell you to go off of your Aleve and use Tylenol, which also builds up in the liver. So what are you to do? If you go off your pain medication, you *hurt*. I know, because that is exactly what happened to me. And besides the fact that Tylenol was destroying my liver, it worked about as well as a glass of water.

The good news is that Rosemary not only detoxifies the liver (reduces the buildup of chemical toxins like the chemicals in Aleve), it also is an anti-inflammatory and a mild pain reliever.

Also, unlike Ibuprofen and other NSAIDs, Rosemary has been successful in easing the pain of ulcers.

Rosemary Tea

1 teaspoon dried Rosemary
1 cup boiling water
Add water to Rosemary.
Let steep for 10-20 minutes
Sip slowly, drinking no more than 1 cup per day. It is potent. Overuse can irritate the stomach.

37

Sage

This recipe is a bit different. Sage has both anti-bacterial and astringent agents, which makes it a terrific topical, gargle or mouthwash. Yes, you can drink Sage Tea. Sipped daily, it helps with chronic digestive complaints.

Because it's mostly a topical, you can use it for acne or other shallow wounds and sores. For acne, wash face with soap and water, blot dry. Using a cotton ball, dab cooled Sage tea over affected area. Do not rinse. In the morning, repeat the process.

As a gargle, add a little lemon to the cooled tea and gargle. As a mouthwash, add a little salt instead.

Cooled Sage Tea, without any additives, makes a natural deodorant. Just put it in a spray bottle and apply when needed.

Sage Tea

1 teaspoon Sage 1 cup boiling water
Pour water over Sage.

Let steep 10-20 minutes. May add lemon to taste or for a gargle.
May add salt for a mouthwash.
Add nothing for a topical astringent or for a deodorant.

38

Summer Savory

Summer Savory is one of those herbs than are terrific in a garden. Not only do they smell wonderful, they're good for both food and medicine. Summer Savory works to help with gastrointestinal issues, alleviates thirst in diabetics and helps during cold season.

Pregnant women should not take Summer Savory.

Gastrointestinal Issues

If you have chronic gastrointestinal problems, look at your diet first. Are you eating too much? Do you have too much sugar in your diet? Are there certain foods you should be avoiding? As you work through those issues, Mild Summer Savory Tea will help. This tea is also mild enough for infants who suffer from colic.

Mild Summer Savory Tea

1 teaspoon Summer Savory

1 cup boiling water

Pour boiling water over chopped herb. Let steep 5-20 minutes. Sip slowly.

Diabetics

Drink Mild Summer Savory Tea to alleviate excessive thirst.

Congestion, Coughs, Sore Throats

When we get to cold and flu season, we need not be victims of viruses. We have an herbal army ready to fight for us. One such soldier is Sage. You can make Strong Summer Savory Tea for all your cold and flu symptoms, even for diarrhea and as an antiseptic to fight germs lingering around the home.

Strong Summer Savory Tea

1 tablespoon Summer Savory
1 cup boiling water
Honey to taste
Poor boiling water over chopped herb. Let steep 20 minutes. Add honey. Sip slowly

To clean the sick room, add a little vinegar, put in a spray bottle, and use to disinfect all surfaces.

Note: Pregnant women should not use Summer Savory

39
Willow Bark

If you buy willow bark, you get the inner bark of the white willow. Other willows also work, such as the red willow which grows in ditches, and never develops into a full-sized tree. It's a shrub that looks like lots of red twigs clumped together in the winter. It's easy to harvest and easy to prepare. Just take fresh, thin willow twigs, remove all the leaves and buds, then shave the soft bark away with a sharp knife. You'll get the outer bark as well, but if you use the tender new branches, it won't matter. You just don't want the wood underneath the bark.

Then you cut the shaved bark into tiny pieces and let dry. Once it's dry, you have a natural pain reliever. However, it's also an NSAID. So if you're sensitive to NSAIDS, use another pain reliever.

Willow Bark Tea is good for soothing menstrual cramps, preventing heart attacks, reducing arthritis and osteoarthritis pain, easing lower back pain, alleviating acne, and eliminating headaches.

Willow Bark Tea
1 teaspoon dried, chopped willow bark
1 cup hot water
Pour water over dried bark.
Let steep for 10 or more minutes.
Strain (or use a tea ball).
Sip slowly.
Dear Reader,

I hope you found this informative and useful. As I've already stated, I'm no doctor, so if you question anything in this book, please go to a professional of your choice.

If you found this helpful, please leave a review. They are more necessary than you know.

AUTHOR'S NOTES

Besides teas, there is much more you can do with healing herbs and Power Foods. Get healthy, stay healthy. Don't let the pharmaceutical industry take your health away.

Dear Reader,

I hope you found this informative and useful. As I've already stated, I'm no doctor, so if you question anything in this book, please go to a professional of your choice.

If you found this helpful, please leave a review. They are more necessary than you know.

MEDICAL DISCLAIMER

The herbal articles are for entertainment and educational purposes only. The author is not a physician and the contents of these articles should not be viewed or taken as medical advice. The views expressed are the opinion of the author and should not be taken as an endorsement of any product or practice. Herbs can and do interact with pharmaceuticals. No herb or herbal product should be taken without consulting a qualified physician. The author disclaims any liability arising directly or indirectly from the use of the information of any product, plant or practice mentioned herein.

ABOUT THE AUTHOR

For years I believed everything my doctor told me, but then a series of things happened. First, I hurt my back. My doctor told me it was just a strained muscle, and never took x-rays. The pain refused to leave, so I did what I always do, I tried to walk it off, never realizing I was exacerbating the problem.

We moved. By that time I could hardly walk and I suffered muscle spasms when I went to bed. I told my new doctor. She suggested stretches. When I told her I couldn't get down on the floor, she asked me why, even after I had told her about my pain. She never suggested x-rays either.

Then one day the pain was so bad I couldn't get out of bed to go to the bathroom during the night. I kept working on it, but the pain was horrible. I was in tears by the time I finally got to the bathroom, even with a walker. I told my husband that I thought I might need to see a chiropractor.

The chiropractor suggested x-rays. So I got them. She then showed me where one vertebrae was twisted, causing all my problems. The x-rays were also sent to my primary physician, who, after seeing the same pictures my chiropractor had seen, told me I had arthritis.

If I had followed my primary physician's advice, I would be in a wheelchair by now.

As I began to research alternative health, my husband came across an article that warned those taking statin drugs that they had a 50% chance of developing Parkinson's Disease if they stopped taking their medication. I was on Simvastatin for high cholesterol.

That began my adventure into herbal medicine.

Dedication

This book is dedicated to the Author of life Who has freely given us the bounty of His world, and Who willingly shares with you His many blessings.

Acknowledgments

The list of those I wish to acknowledge for making this book possible is long. But I must honor at least two people. I must give credit to my husband, who always gives me the time I need to write. I also need to give a big note of thanks to Christy Martinez, my beta reader. I have waited a long time for this friendship, because she is interested in the very subjects I write.

ISBN-10 : 1537040049

ISBN-13 : 978-1537040042

OTHER BOOKS BY MAMA PREPPER

Herbal/Survival:
39 Healthy Teas You Can Make at Home
Healing Herbs from Your Kitchen
Mama Prepper's Herbal Garden
Mama's Medicines – Growing Your Backyard Apothecary

* 9 7 8 1 5 3 7 0 4 0 0 4 2 *